the **little book** of
weight loss
habits
...and how to build them

© Weight Loss Resources 2017

Published by: Weight Loss Resources Ltd, 2C Flag Business Exchange, Vicarage Farm Road, Peterborough PE1 5TX.

Tel: 01733 345592

www.weightlossresources.co.uk

ISBN 978-1-904512-18-9

Printed and bound in the UK

Contents

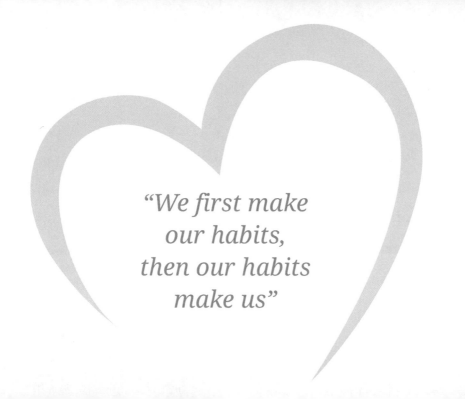

*"We first make
our habits,
then our habits
make us"*

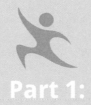

Part 1:

Why You Should Focus on Habits if You Want to Lose Weight

"If you do what you've always done, you'll get what you've always got"

The habits we have tend to make some kind of sense:

We brush our teeth because we want to keep them, go to work because we need the money, eat takeaway because we're busy and snacks because they're there.

Habits help us quickly and easily navigate through daily routine without having to think about it too much.

But the very mindlessness that makes habits useful, works against us when it comes to what, why and when we eat. Without thinking, we'll:

- Eat more food if a larger portion is served
- Eat high calorie low quality food because that's what's in the vending machine
- Keep eating if the bowl of snacks is within arms' reach, even when we don't feel hungry

We need these habits, because deciding between alternatives every time we do something is a hassle. So we rely on what's around us rather than making conscious choices. We go with the flow.

This presents a problem when it comes to our eating habits. The decision making shortcuts (i.e., habits) we use, are tending to make us fat.

So if we want to weigh less we need to take back control. Stop relying on external cues to make our eating decisions for us, and start consciously making our own.

If we consciously make our own decisions, we can make them so that they are leading us toward our weight goals, rather than further and further away.

Of course our environment is not entirely to blame for our tendency to overeat. We use food for a variety of different reasons, e.g.:

- To celebrate
- To relieve boredom
- To make us feel happier

The problem is that eating for reasons other than physical hunger, especially if we do it regularly, will also make us fat.

Excess weight comes from eating more calories than you need, whether that's due to mindless eating, emotion based eating, or a combination of both.

This little book will help you make new habits to bring what you eat, and what you do, back into line with what your body really needs. So you can lose weight for the long term.

How to Use This Book

All the habits in this book are proven to be effective for weight loss, practical, and simple to apply. (Note we didn't say easy!)

Some will have small effects week-to-week, but make a real difference when viewed over a longer period. These habits tend to be the easiest to build.

Others will have bigger effects, i.e., see it on the scales week-to-week weight loss. These habits tend to require a little more effort.

Which you choose to start with will depend on how much time and energy you have available to work on project you, what your goals are, and how quickly you'd like to reach them.

To give you an idea of how much each habit could help you, we've estimated the weight loss potential of adopting a particular habit for a period of three months.

Bear in mind that some habits address similar issues to others, but in a different way – so you can't just add up all the weight loss estimates and assume they'll help you lose 20lbs a month!

The estimates are for guidance, to help you assess the impact an individual habit could have on you.

Here are some examples:

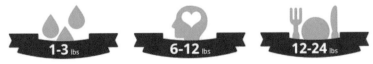

Look out for them throughout the book to help you choose where to start.

How to Create a New Habit that Sticks

We've all had occasions in the past when we have intended to lose weight, and failed to make it happen.

There's a good reason for this.

Whilst having an intention, or even a goal, is important. It's not enough to get us to take the steps necessary to achieve it.

It doesn't give us the cues and tactics we need to use in everyday life. It doesn't help us to create new habits, so we end up falling back on the old ones.

As the saying goes:

"If you do what you've always done, you'll get what you've always got."

Use If/When – Then

If/When – Then statements enable us to take an intention or goal, and turn it into practical steps we can take in order to achieve it. We then take these steps over and over again until they become automatic – a habit.

Some examples:

"<u>If</u> I am going be eating lunch in my office, <u>then</u> I will take a packed lunch to work."

 "<u>When</u> I order a meal from McDonalds, <u>then</u> I will order a side salad with my burger rather than fries."

"<u>When</u> I'm going from place to place throughout my day, <u>then</u> I will use every opportunity to take the stairs rather than the lift."

You need to make an **if/when – then** statement for each of the habits you choose to develop to help you reach your goal.

Each habit has example statements to get you started. Plus there are progress charts at the back so you can write your own **if/when – then** statements, and keep a record of how you're doing.

When you first get started, choose habits that seem like they would be quite easy for you to fit into your life.

Early wins will help to build your confidence and show you that making changes isn't going to ruin your life!

Bear in mind that it very likely won't be all plain sailing, especially when you first get started.

You'll have days when some or all of your if/when - then tactics get buried under other stuff. It doesn't mean that you've failed - the important thing is to get right back to it the next day.

Good luck!

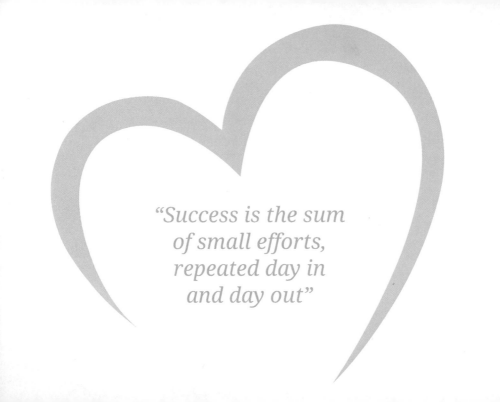

"Success is the sum
of small efforts,
repeated day in
and day out"

Part 2:

Food Related Habits

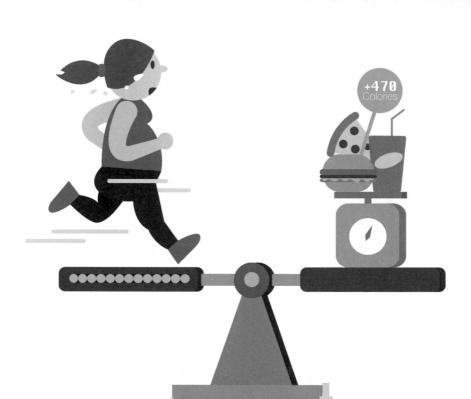

Calorie Balance

Your habits with regard to food are, not surprisingly, the most important when it comes to how much you weigh.

This is because all foods (and many drinks) contain calories, and your body essentially makes fat out of those calories it doesn't need to keep you going in your day-to-day life.

In order to maintain your weight at a steady level you need to eat as many calories as you burn, and no more.

In order to lose weight, you need to eat fewer calories than you burn. That is, you need to create a calorie deficit.

When you don't feed your body enough calories to meet your daily needs, it draws energy from its reserves and you lose weight.

Creating a Calorie Deficit

A pound of fat contains around 3500 calories. So if you want to lose a pound a week, you need to eat 3500 calories less than you burn. That is, create a calorie deficit of 3500 per week.

Therefore you need to eat 500 calories a day less than you burn, to create a deficit big enough to lose a pound in a week.

The UK health department says that on average, a woman needs 2000 calories and a man needs 2500 calories per day.

This is a useful rule of thumb, but bear in mind that there can be wide differences between individuals, depending on how active they are, their age, height and weight.

Average Calorie Allowances to Lose Weight

	Men	Women
Maintain Weight	2500	2000
Lose ½lb a week	2250	1750
Lose 1lb a week	2000	1500
Lose 1½lb a week	1750	1250
Lose 2lb a week	1500	1000

To get a more accurate idea of your own calorie needs, you can do a free trial at weightlossresources.co.uk and it will be worked out for you.

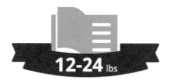

12-24 lbs

New Habit - Keep a Food Diary

Research shows that people who record what they eat lose twice as much weight as those who just try healthy eating and activity.

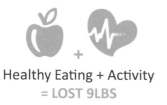

Healthy Eating + Activity
= LOST 9LBS

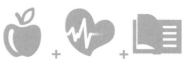

Healthy Eating + Activity + Food Diary
= LOST 20LBS

That's **11** extra pounds, just from keeping a food diary.

Make it Easy

There are various options for keeping food diary.

To make it quick and easy, use your mobile phone, tablet or any computer. The wlr food diary enables you to use all 3 devices easily, and the food database is designed for UK users.

Alternatively, you could keep a notebook style diary, and write everything down through the day. Then use a calorie counting reference book such as the Calorie Carb & Fat Bible, to look up and tot up your calories.

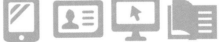

Make "Food Diary" Your Habit

When are you going to fill your food diary in?

Just after every time you eat? After dinner? When you're watching TV?

Think about what would suit you best. If you spend a lot of time on your mobile, the first option could be good for you. If you're very busy throughout the day, in the evening could work better for you.

"If I eat something, I will record it in my food diary straight away"

 "When I have finished eating dinner, I will record everything I have eaten today in my food diary"

"In the evening when I'm watching TV, I will fill in my food diary"

When Would You Do Yours?

	If *or* When	
HABIT	Then	

Pre-empt Problems

Try to think of issues that would stop you from following your if/when-then plan, and decide what you'll do in advance.

"If my wi-fi's down, then I'll note everything down and fill in my diary tomorrow."

"If I'm going out tonight, then I'll keep up with the diary through the day and finish it off in the morning."

Progressing Your Food Diary Habit

Getting into the habit of logging every day is the absolute best thing you can do to get long term results.

Don't worry too much about staying within a strict calorie allowance to start with. Focus on embedding the diary habit.

Then you could try making sure you stay below your maintenance calorie level, or experimenting with different rates of loss to see what level you think you can cope with.

When you have a decided on a calorie allowance you can live with, that is lower than the calories you would need to maintain your current weight, stick with it and start getting really great results.

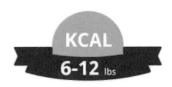

New Habit - Trim Your Calorie Allowance Gobblers

We've all got them, high calorie favourites that can blow a calorie allowance out of the water.

The trick here is to replace or reduce rather than deny. Denying yourself food you like is not a very successful way of trying to break a habit.

In fact research shows that trying to break a habit simply by saying you won't do it anymore, is the least effective way to make it happen.

Even worse, forbidding yourself from eating a food you like can have a rebound effect, leading you to want the food even more.

Spot the Difference

I'm not going to eat pizza any more	VS	**When I want pizza for dinner, then I'll have half a pizza and a side salad**
I'm going to give up chocolate	VS	**If I really want some chocolate, then I'll have a funsize bar**
I'm going to quit eating Doughnuts	VS	**When I want an afternoon snack, then I will eat a light cereal bar**

Make "Trimming" Your Habit

Think about the foods, and drinks, you consume regularly that are high in calories. Especially look at those that seem to have become a bit of a habit. Jot a couple of ideas down now.

HABIT	If *or* When	
	Then	

HABIT	If *or* When	
	Then	

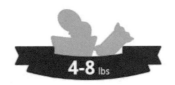

4-8 lbs

New Habit - Make Yourself a Snack Box (or Two)

If you're a regular snacker, this will really help.

The best thing about having a snack box is that you always have something in stock that's not going to damage your weight loss goals.

Plus it saves your mind the strife of having to make tricky decisions about snacks throughout the day. Not to mention the seduction of the sweet counter.

Find some snack foods that you like, that don't cost you too many calories.

Impose calories per portion limit for items that are allowed into the snack box.

Say, no more than 10% of your daily calorie allowance per snack. So, if your allowance is 1200 calories, each snack in the box would be 120 calories or less.

Remember you can always break things down into smaller portions, so that they fit within your limit. Just make sure they are packaged into portions of the right size before they go into the box.

Take an item or two from the snack box with you if you are going to be at work, or out somewhere, and are likely to want a snack. This saves you from going to the vending machine or coffee shop, both of which are full of high calorie temptations.

It's worth spending some time researching what kinds of things you could put in your box. Two boxes, if you want one for the fridge and one for the cupboard.

You could have a browse around a supermarket or look online, wlr regularly publishes food ideas articles and information about new food products.

The important thing is to make sure that everything is in calorie-counted portions. For example, if you like to eat nuts, or dried fruits, portion them up into little bags containing the right number of calories.

You'll probably also find it helpful to get some small, airtight plastic containers for holding fresh foods.

Snack box Ideas

- Low calorie cereal bars
- Fruit, single pieces or fruit salads
- Small bags of crisps (the 20-25g ones from a multi-pack)
- Vegetable sticks and dip
- Low fat yoghurts
- Low calorie hot-chocolate sachets
- 20-30g portions of nuts
- 30-40g portions of olives
- Fun size chocolate bars, or full size cut into portions and wrapped separately
- Cuppa soups
- Crispbread and low fat cream cheese

Make "Snack Box" Your Habit

Keep your snacks put away somewhere. This strategy won't work very well if you're dipping into the box all day. Decide on a daily snacks number that seems right for you, and stick within it.

"When I have my after-work snack, then I'll take it from my snackbox."

"If I want a snack when I'm watching TV, then I'll take it from my snackbox."

HABIT		
If *or* When		
Then		

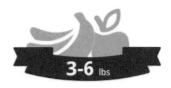

3-6 lbs

New Habit - Have a Fruit Bowl

If you don't fancy making up a snack box, make it easy and convenient for yourself to snack on fab-for-your-figure fruit.

Research has shown that keeping an attractive bowl of fruit in a highly visible and convenient location, (like the kitchen side) makes it much more likely that you'll increase your fruit intake.

Not only is snacking on fruit better for your figure than high-sugar snacks, it will also satisfy you for longer.

"If I want a snack, when I am at home, I will choose something from the fruit bowl."

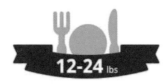

12-24 lbs

New Habit - Practice Portion Control

Most of us haven't a clue what the recommended serving sizes of our favourite breakfast cereals look like. Our 'standard' serving size is whatever amount we pour into the bowl.

It turns out that quite a lot of us eat 1.5 to 2 times the amount of a recommended cereal serving without ever realising. We may even glance at the calorie info on the pack and be lulled into a completely false sense of security - "not too many calories in that".

Cereal is just one common example of portion distortion. In fact, most people under-estimate most portions - especially large ones!

Make it Easy

It doesn't matter so much if you're eating vegetables or fruit, or drinking no-added-sugar squash. You wouldn't be causing any damage if you underestimated a serving of steamed broccoli, which has only 24 calories in a large, 100g portion.

Other foods and drinks do make a difference. Funnily enough, fruit juice is one that often trips people up. At around 46 calories per 100ml, a normal 250ml glass of orange juice is 115 calories.

The higher calorie a food or drink, the more important that you measure it. Fats and oils are at the top of the tree at around 9 calories per gram.

If you want to lose weight, you need to make sure you're in control of your portions.

If you don't have them already, get yourself some easy to use, easy to clean digital kitchen scales.

Digital because the weight shown is not open to interpretation like a dial is. If you're still using a dial it's probably time to trade it in.

You'll also want a range of measuring spoons, cups and jugs. These items can be bought for a few pounds and are well worth the money for the time, effort and excess calories they'll save you.

Some small light-weight plastic bowls to contain food you want to weigh will be handy to use with your scales, particularly if you have the type with a flat platform.

Simply weigh the bowl without the food, then with the food. Subtract the weight of the bowl from the total to get your food weight.

Make "Portion Control" Your Habit

"When there's food that I don't know the weight of, then I will weigh it before I eat it."

 "If my breakfast cereal pours straight from the box, then I will weigh it."

"If I'm eating in a restaurant, I will try to accurately estimate the weight of each food on the plate."

Try your Own:

HABIT	If *or* When	
	Then	

New Habit - Drink Water

Drinking water is probably the easiest thing you can do to help your weight loss along. Numerous studies have shown that those who drink plenty of water lose more weight, and generally weigh less, than those who don't.

According to research, there are a number of possible reasons why water helps weight loss. Top of the list are:

- If you're well-hydrated, you're less likely to mistake thirst for hunger and eat something you don't really need.

- It takes a few extra calories for your body to warm up chilled or iced water.
- Water can temporarily fill your stomach for zero calories

Try to get 3 large glasses a day. Iced if you can, add no-sugar flavour if you're not keen on plain water. Fizzy water is also fine.

Whilst this habit is easy to do, it's also easy to forget.

Increase your chances of success by scheduling your water for times when you would normally eat or drink. Or tie drinking a glass of water with something else you do habitually every day.

Drinking cold water 20-30 minutes before meals has additional weight loss benefits because of the energy you expend to warm it up, and the effect of filling your stomach before you eat.

Make "Water" Your Habit

The best way to do this is three times a day, before meals. So your if/when – then statement could be as simple as:

"When it's 30 minutes before a meal, I will drink a glass of water."

Don't worry if you don't remember until five minutes before your meal. Still drink the water.

If you're not keen on the idea of water before meals, try a statement that would work for you.

HABIT		
	If *or* When	
	Then	

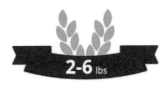

New Habit - Fill Up on Fibre

Recognised as a hero food component by Audrey Eyton in her best-selling F Plan Diet, things have been pretty quiet on the fibre front lately.

But fibre is still as much of a friend to would be weight losers as it always was. It fills you up, and keeps everything moving along as it should.

Foods high in fibre add bulk to your meals and snacks, helping you to feel more satisfied on fewer calories. Plus there's the added bonus that fibre rich foods are also full of essential, health protecting nutrients.

Most of us tend not to get enough fibre, so take it gently - aiming for 20g a day to start with, moving up to 25g a day after a few weeks.

Fibre Rich Foods

The following foods will help you bump up fibre intake:

- Wholemeal, granary or wholegrain bread or rolls
- Potatoes, baked or boiled in their skins
- Beans and peas – including baked beans
- Fresh and dried fruits
- Wholegrain breakfast cereals such as Weetabix, Branflakes, Shreddies, porridge oats
- Nuts and seeds
- Any and all vegetables
- Brown rice and pasta
- Quinoa, other whole grains and wholemeal flour
- Chick peas, lentils and other pulses

Make "Fibre" Your Habit

"If I am going to eat bread, then I will eat wholemeal bread."

 "When I have breakfast, I will eat high fibre cereal."

"When I eat dinner, I will have at least 2 different vegetables with it."

How could you get more fibre into your life? Have a go at a statement for yourself.

HABIT	If *or* When	
	Then	

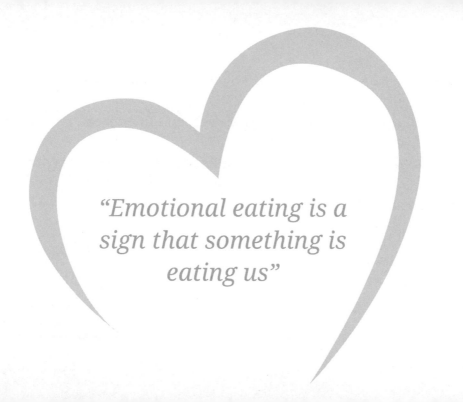

"Emotional eating is a sign that something is eating us"

Part 3:

Emotion Related Habits

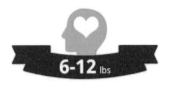

6-12 lbs

New Habit - Get to Know Your Hunger

Are you hungry or do you really want a hug, a bit of peace, or something interesting to do?

When your body physically needs something, it sends a message to your brain. Like when you go to the loo - your bladder tells your brain it needs to empty – you find a loo.

Hunger should work in the same way. Your stomach rumble sends a message to your brain that you're hungry – you find some food.

The problem comes when we eat in response to some other stimulus, that could be as simple as boredom or as complex as needing a hug.

Physical or Emotional? Know the Difference

Physical Hunger	Emotional Hunger
Builds gradually	Develops suddenly
Strikes below the neck *(e.g., growling stomach)*	Above the neck *(e.g., a "taste" for ice cream)*
Occurs several hours after a meal	Unrelated to time
Goes away when full	Persists despite fullness
Eating leads to feeling of satisfaction	Eating leads to guilt and shame

Think Thin, Be Thin Hales and Hemering 2004

Knowing your hunger, and responding accordingly, could turn out to be a game changer for you if you often eat when you're not physically hungry.

It's not the easiest habit to acquire, mainly because it's hard to remember to do it before you go to eat something. But it can be done with a little practice and will pay you dividends in terms of weight loss.

After all, what's the point of eating something, if eating isn't going to solve problem. The only problem eating can solve is physical hunger.

You'll be far better off finding other solutions to whatever issues are causing you to eat for comfort, distraction or other emotional reasons.

Eating when you're not really hungry just leaves you with another problem to solve.

The Hunger Questions

Asking yourself the following two questions will help you to determine if your current hunger is physical or emotional.

Remember to ask them before you eat.

Am I suddenly hungry, or has the feeling been building over a while?

Is my stomach rumbling, or do I have a taste for something?

The answers to these questions will tell you if your hunger is emotional or physical.

If you're not sure, ask yourself if you 'should' be hungry – based on when you had your last meal and what you ate.

When you are able to recognise the difference, and you will if you practice, you can start building habits to overcome emotional eating.

Make "Knowing Hunger" Your Habit

There are two parts to developing this habit effectively,

 "If feel like eating, before I eat, I will ask myself the hunger questions."

Develop this habit of asking the hunger questions first. You may not find making this diagnosis so easy to start with. You might not be sure, your emotions may over-ride your physical feelings.

But stick with it, it's not so hard to ask yourself a question. You'll soon have a better understanding of what's going on.

Building the habit of asking the hunger questions, and doing your best to answer them honestly, is the foundation of being able to do something about it. You need to take a second step to have a real effect on your weight.

Once you can recognise if you are physically hungry or not, you should follow on with a statement something like this:

"If I feel like eating when I'm not physically hungry, then I will have a glass of flavoured water."

"If I'm feeling hungry because I'm fed up, then I will light some candles and have a fragrant, bubbly bath."

Think of an alternative that you could do, that would work to quiet your own non-physical hunger.

HABIT	If *or* When	
	Then	

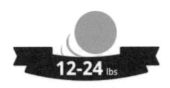

New Habit - Bounce Back Quickly

Lots of people start a new 'diet' almost every week, because of all or nothing thinking. They have a bad day and eat more than they planned and their diet is "ruined".

They'll have to start over, maybe next week. And since "the diet starts Monday", they might as well make the most of the eating opportunities over the next few days.

Some people get caught in this trap for years – feeling like they are 'always on a diet' whilst they slowly keep on gaining weight.

The worst thing you can do when you're trying to lose weight and you go 'off plan', is surrender to all or nothing thinking.

It can go something like this:

"OMG I stuffed myself silly/drunk myself stupid/binged on a packet of biscuits. I won't lose any weight this week, I might as well give up."

Or:

"OMG, I ate way too much at lunchtime. There's no way I'll be able to stick to my calorie allowance today, I might as well give up."

You should forgive yourself immediately and get back on track at the earliest possible opportunity. If you have an over-indulgent lunch, get back on track by dinner. If you go over the top on a night out (or a night in raiding the fridge) get back on track the next morning.

Make "Bouncing Back Quickly" Your Habit

"When there is an occasion where I eat or drink more than I really wanted to, then I'll get back to my new habits before my next meal."

"If I have a bad day and blow my calorie allowance, then I will get back on track the next day."

What could you do to prevent yourself becoming a victim of all or nothing thinking?

HABIT	If *or* When	
	Then	

Part 4:
Lifestyle Related Habits

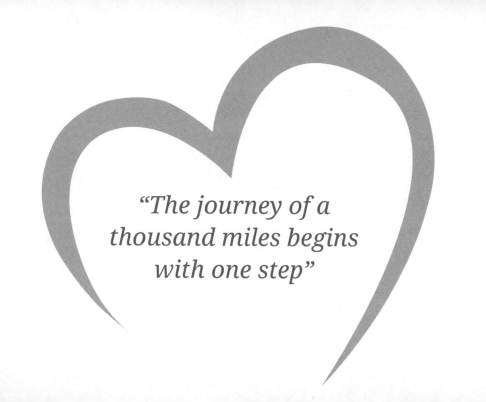

"The journey of a thousand miles begins with one step"

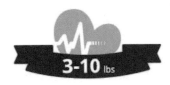

Habit - Get 10 Minutes Exercise a Day

You may think that 10 minutes exercise a day is not enough to make a difference. But it is enough to start building a habit. And enough to start burning some extra calories.

When you're beginning to make this new habit, keep it as simple as possible. Something super simple like...

Walk out the door and keep going for 5 minutes

Then walk back

Do it as briskly as you can and you've done your 10 minutes today.

Make "Exercise" Your Habit

Think about the times you could possibly fit it in 10 minutes to take a walk. The 'best' time to exercise is always the time that suits you best.

"If I am at home in the evening, then I will do 10 minutes exercise before dinner."

"When I'm on my lunch break, then I will do 10 minutes exercise after lunch."

HABIT	If *or* When	
	Then	

Make Your Excuses in Advance

When it is raining, then I will take an umbrella

When it is dark, then I will take a torch

If it is windy, then I'll cover my ears with a hat

When it is cold, then I'll wrap up warm

If I am busy, then I'll just do 5 minutes

When I am tired, then I'll do a gentle session

If I can't be bothered, then I'll put my headphones on and move to the beat

Keep On Moving On

Once you're confident with your 10 minutes a day exercise habit, step it up a little. You could try adding an extra 10 minutes a day on 3 or 4 days a week to start with.

You can keep it as simple as extending your Walk Out Walk Back by 10 minutes. Or you could try something different:

- Cycling
- Swimming
- A workout from a book, YouTube or DVD

Eventually getting to 30 minutes, 5 times a week, will be great for your weight loss and your health.

Any activity that gets you moving at more effort than normal will work. Aim for a 3-5 on the effort scale.

Exercise Effort Scale

0	Nothing at all
0.5	Just noticeable
1	Very light
2	Light
3	Moderate
4	Somewhat heavy
5	Heavy
6	
7	Very heavy
8	
9	
10	Very, very heavy
**	Maximal

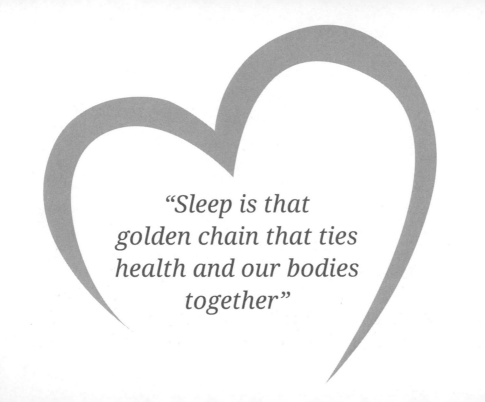

"Sleep is that golden chain that ties health and our bodies together"

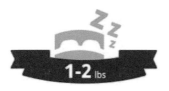

New Habit - Get Enough Sleep

Numerous studies in recent years have explored the relationship between sleep duration and weight loss. And the almost unanimous conclusion is that lack of sleep contributes to weight gain.

The main reasons for this appear to be:

- Eating more sugary snacks and refined carbohydrates, possibly to provide extra energy to tired brains
- Sluggish metabolism and reduced energy expenditure
- More impulsivity, so more likelihood of snacking
- Hormonal changes leading to increased appetite

This habit has a low potential weight loss score because it's difficult to tell how much difference it would make in a wide range of individual circumstances.

However, if you find yourself sitting up late at night snacking or drinking, it could be a major contributory factor in why you have gained weight. And, in all likelihood, you will continue to gain if you don't make some changes.

In these circumstances, getting a minimum 7 hours a night could make a much bigger difference to your weight over a 3-month period.

Feeling tired also has a contributory effect on our mood. So lack of sleep could very likely contribute to the problem of eating in response to non-physical hunger.

Make "Sleep" Your Habit

"If I need to get up at 7am, then I will go to bed before midnight."

"When it is 11.30pm, then I will start getting ready for bed."

Plan to do something like this, adjusted to suit your own daily pattern. Even if you don't think you'll be able to sleep, go to bed and read a book, and let yourself fall asleep when you're ready. It can take some time to change your sleeping patterns.

HABIT	If *or* When	
	Then	

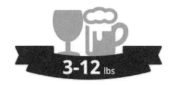

3-12 lbs

New Habit - Practice Alcohol Control

At 7.1 per gram, alcohol has nearly twice as many calories as sugar or protein. This means that a small (25ml) of 40% abv spirits contains around 55 calories.

Have 2 or 3 of these small drinks a day and you've got 50,000 extra calories a year to burn off if you don't want to gain weight.

Or, to put it another way, you'll gain around a stone in a year if you don't eat less to make up for the alcohol calories.

If you're a beer or wine drinker the numbers only get worse.

That's not to say that you can't have a drink and lose weight. But you do need to control the amount that you drink.

You can do that by having alcohol free days, or by measuring and limiting your drinks every day.

Calories in Popular Alcoholic Drinks

Red Wine	1 med glass/175ml	146 cals
Draught Beer	1 pint/568ml	182 cals
Cider	1 pint/568ml	205 cals
Vodka	1 shot/25ml	56 cals

Make "Alcohol Control" Your Habit

"If I have a drink after work, I will use a measure when I pour it."

"If I go to the pub, then I will drink only half pints."

"When I open a bottle of wine, then I will pour one glass, seal the bottle and put it away."

You could try drinking water or diet soda between alcoholic drinks when you're out, or being alcohol free on 5 days a week.

HABIT	If *or* When	
	Then	

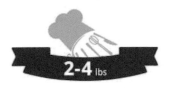

New Habit - Cook at Home

People who eat home cooked food most nights of the week, consume up to 140 less calories a day than those who rely on ready meals, restaurants and takeaways.

That amounts to over 50,000 calories in a year - the equivalent of 14lbs, a whole stone!

How easy it will be to build this habit will depend on your circumstances. But if you don't currently eat home-cooked food often, a stone in a year has got to be worth a bit of effort.

You don't suddenly have to turn into Master Chef

Everyone's short of time these days. Look online for quick and easy evening meals, or get yourself a few recipe books. The wlr recipe database has thousands of recipes that you can search and sort by ingredient, calorie value, etc.

The key to easy evening meals is a little pre-planning. Make a rough list of meal ideas for the week, and take the list when you go shopping.

Get double the quantities, or more, for meals that can go in the freezer, so you don't have to start from scratch every night.

Make "Cooking" Your Habit

"When it is Sunday morning, then I will cook 2 different meals to go in the freezer."

"On Tuesday evenings, I will try out new recipes."

"When I go shopping this week, then I'll make sure I plan for quick mid-week dinners."

What, how, when and even if you cook will be dependent on your circumstances. What's a statement that could work for you?

HABIT	If or When	
	Then	

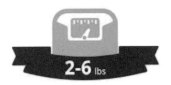

2-6 lbs

Habit - Weigh Yourself Frequently

Recent studies have shown a positive link between how often a person steps on the scales and how much weight they lose or, importantly, don't gain. This is particularly the case when they are able to record and view their results in graphical form.

The same holds true for people who have lost weight. They are more likely to maintain their weight loss successfully if they are frequent self-weighers.

So what does frequent mean?

In the studies referred to above people weighed in at least three times a week, and some weighed themselves daily.

It appears that there are three main reasons why weighing yourself frequently could help with weight control:

- Viewing your weight graph over a period of time provides feedback enabling you to make a better connection with your own energy balance (i.e. calories consumed versus calories burned).
- The number on the scale may act as either positive or negative reinforcement. Seeing a loss at your morning weigh-in could positively reinforce healthy choices you made on the previous day.
- On the other hand, a gain in the morning could put a negative light on last night's fast food blowout.
- Weighing-in in the morning, and seeing a graph, may strengthen your resolve in the face of social and environmental cues associated with eating.

Make "Frequent Weighing" Your Habit

Try to weigh yourself first thing in the morning as this is when your body weight will be most consistent from day-to-day.

 "When I wake up in the morning, after I've been to the loo, then I will weigh myself and record my weight."

"If it's a weekday, then I will weigh myself when I get up."

HABIT	If *or* When	
	Then	

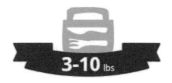

3-10 lbs

Habit - Plan Your Work-Day Lunches

Packing your own lunch gives you a lot more control over calories than grabbing something from the local coffee shop or fast food outlet.

This is especially true if you pop out to pick up lunch just before you eat it, when you're likely to be feeling hungry.

It's probably too much to ask yourself to watch the calories, when your tummy's rumbling and the sights and smells of tempting food are all around you. You're making it hard work.

You can make your packup every bit as good as something from a takeaway and, when it comes to pre-packed sandwiches, probably a whole lot better.

Of course you don't have to stick to boring old sandwiches in your lunchbox, you can make it much more tasty, interesting and satisfying. Here are some ideas:

- Soup, either home-made or a variety you enjoy from a tin or chilled pack. If you don't have access to a microwave at work, use a flask.
- Wraps, pittas and bagels all make a welcome change from the sliced white bread with ham routine. Go for whole grain versions and top off your main ingredients with plenty of crunchy salad.
- Leftovers from last night's dinner can feel quite luxurious when eaten at your desk or in the lunch room. Try to serve in a different way, or with different accompaniments to keep it interesting.

Make "A Pack Up" Your Habit

The most important part of making this habit work is planning – making sure you have the ingredients, and the time to get them into your lunch box.

"When I have finished dinner, then I will make my packed lunch for the next day."

"If I am shopping, then I will make sure I buy food for my lunches."

What could work for you?

HABIT	If *or* When	
	Then	

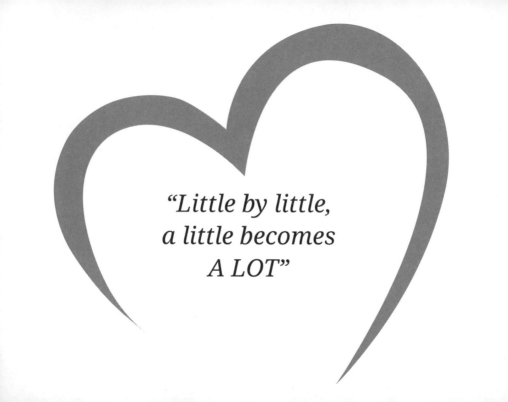

*"Little by little,
a little becomes
A LOT"*

Part 5:
Progress Charts

| **HABIT 1** | If *or* When | |
| | Then | |

| **HABIT 2** | If *or* When | |
| | Then | |

| **HABIT 3** | If *or* When | |
| | Then | |

Wk 1	Mon	Tues	Weds	Thurs	Fri	Sat	Sun
1							
2							
3							

Wk 2	Mon	Tues	Weds	Thurs	Fri	Sat	Sun
1							
2							
3							

Wk 3	Mon	Tues	Weds	Thurs	Fri	Sat	Sun
1							
2							
3							

Wk 4	Mon	Tues	Weds	Thurs	Fri	Sat	Sun
1							
2							
3							

Wk 5	Mon	Tues	Weds	Thurs	Fri	Sat	Sun
1							
2							
3							

Wk 6	Mon	Tues	Weds	Thurs	Fri	Sat	Sun
1							
2							
3							

Wk 7	Mon	Tues	Weds	Thurs	Fri	Sat	Sun
1							
2							
3							

Wk 8	Mon	Tues	Weds	Thurs	Fri	Sat	Sun
1							
2							
3							

Wk 9	Mon	Tues	Weds	Thurs	Fri	Sat	Sun
1							
2							
3							

Wk 10	Mon	Tues	Weds	Thurs	Fri	Sat	Sun
1							
2							
3							

Wk 11	Mon	Tues	Weds	Thurs	Fri	Sat	Sun
1							
2							
3							

Wk 12	Mon	Tues	Weds	Thurs	Fri	Sat	Sun
1							
2							
3							

About Weight Loss Resources

The focus at wlr is on providing tools to help you get calories into balance and make sustainable habit changes. All wrapped up in a warm, kind-hearted community with a wealth of experience and practical advice.

We don't advocate strange diets. In fact, to us, there's no such thing as a forbidden food.

We've been around a long time, so we know that whatever you do to lose weight, it has to work with your lifestyle.

That's why we offer the most comprehensive tools and databases for weight loss in the UK. And we're constantly improving them based on the evidence of what works for weight loss.

The easiest way to see how wlr could help you is to take a free trial at www.weightlossresources.co.uk

Need Some Help?

The infamous Weight Loss Resources Helpteam are on hand seven days a week. You just have to give them a call, send them an email or message, to get a prompt, understanding and helpful response.

Email helpteam@weightlossresources.co.uk

Phone 01733 345592

Or log in to the message boards at Weight Loss Resources. Post on the Helpteam message board or send us a private message.